How To Manage Schizophrenia

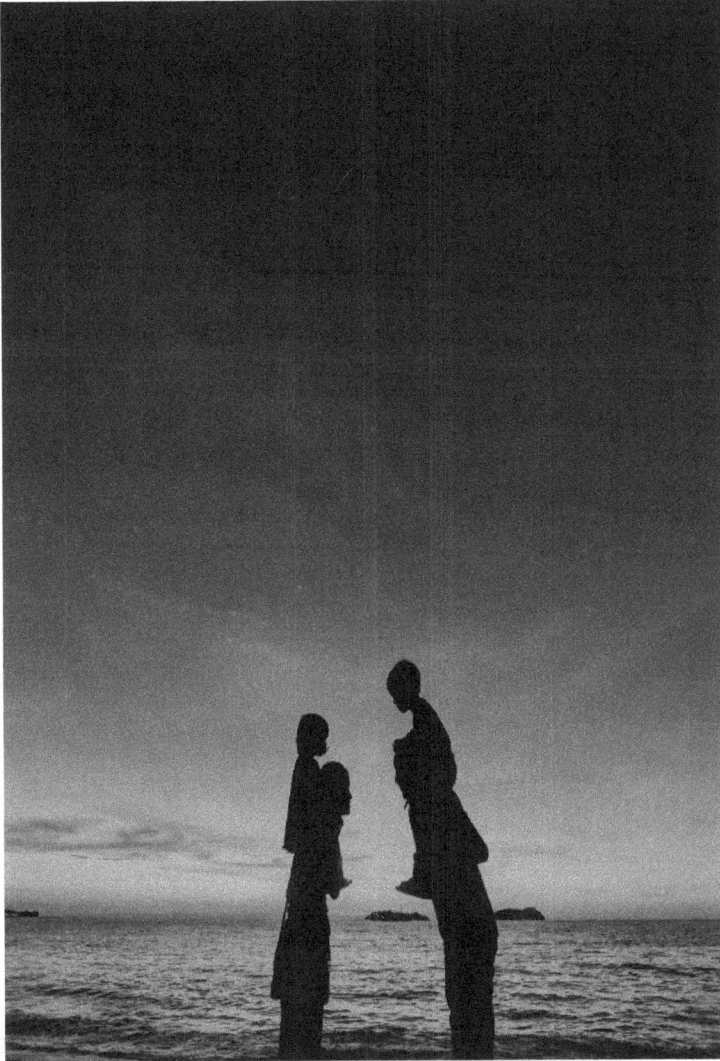

A Family's Guide to Navigating the Challenges

Chapter 1

Understanding Schizophrenia

What is Schizophrenia?

Schizophrenia is a complex and often misunderstood mental health disorder that affects how a person thinks, feels, and behaves. It is characterized by symptoms such as delusions, hallucinations, disorganized thinking, and difficulty with social interactions. While the exact cause of schizophrenia is not yet fully understood, it is believed to be a combination of genetic, environmental, and neurobiological factors.

People with schizophrenia may experience a variety of symptoms that can vary in severity and frequency. These symptoms can make it challenging for individuals to function in daily life and may require ongoing treatment and support.

This publication is intended to provide educational information for the reader on the covered subjects. It is not intended to take the place of personalized medical counseling, diagnosis, and treatment from a trained healthcare professional.

ISBN 978-1-998740-22-2 (Paperback)

Printed and bound in USA
Published by Loons Press

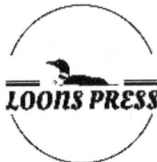

LOONS PRESS

Table Of Contents

It is important for family members and loved ones to educate themselves about schizophrenia and its symptoms in order to better understand and support their loved one who has been diagnosed with the disorder.

Managing schizophrenia can be a lifelong journey that requires a combination of medication, therapy, and support from family and mental health professionals. It is important for individuals with schizophrenia to work closely with their healthcare team to develop a treatment plan that addresses their specific needs and goals.

This may include regular medication management, therapy sessions, and support groups to help cope with the challenges of living with schizophrenia.

Family members can play a crucial role in supporting their loved one with schizophrenia by providing emotional support, helping with medication management, and encouraging them to stay on track with their treatment plan.

It is important for families to communicate openly and honestly with each other about the challenges they may face and to work together to find solutions that work for everyone involved. By working together, families can help their loved one with schizophrenia live a fulfilling and meaningful life.

In conclusion, schizophrenia is a complex and challenging disorder that requires ongoing support and understanding from family members and mental health professionals.

By educating themselves about the symptoms and treatment options for schizophrenia, families can better support their loved one in managing their condition and living a fulfilling life. With the right support and resources, individuals with schizophrenia can lead happy and productive lives.

Common Symptoms of Schizophrenia

Schizophrenia is a complex mental health condition that can be challenging to understand and manage. One of the key aspects of supporting someone with schizophrenia is recognizing and understanding the common symptoms associated with the disorder.

By being aware of these symptoms, individuals and their families can better navigate the challenges that come with managing schizophrenia.

One of the most common symptoms of schizophrenia is hallucinations. These can manifest in various forms, such as hearing voices that others cannot hear or seeing things that are not there. Hallucinations can be distressing and disorienting for the individual experiencing them, and it is important for family members to provide support and understanding during these episodes.

Another common symptom of schizophrenia is delusions. These are false beliefs that are not based in reality, such as believing that one is being followed or that their thoughts are being controlled by external forces. Delusions can be difficult to challenge or rationalize with the individual, but offering a non-judgmental and supportive environment can help them feel safe and understood.

Disorganized thinking and speech are also common symptoms of schizophrenia. This can manifest in the form of jumbled thoughts, difficulty expressing oneself clearly, or jumping from one topic to another without a logical connection. It is important for family members to be patient and understanding when communicating with someone experiencing disorganized thinking, and to help them stay focused and organized in their thoughts and speech.

Negative symptoms, such as a lack of motivation, social withdrawal, and difficulty expressing emotions, are also common in schizophrenia. These symptoms can make it challenging for individuals to engage in daily activities, maintain relationships, or seek help when needed.

Family members can provide support by encouraging and assisting with activities of daily living, offering companionship and social support, and helping the individual access appropriate mental health services.

Overall, understanding the common symptoms of schizophrenia is essential for individuals and their families to effectively manage the challenges that come with the disorder. By being aware of these symptoms and providing support and understanding, families can help their loved ones navigate the complexities of schizophrenia and work towards better mental health and well-being.

Causes of Schizophrenia

Schizophrenia is a complex and often misunderstood mental health condition that affects millions of people worldwide. While the exact cause of schizophrenia is not fully understood, researchers believe that a combination of genetic, environmental, and neurochemical factors play a role in the development of the disorder.

One of the primary causes of schizophrenia is believed to be genetics. Studies have shown that individuals with a family history of schizophrenia are at a higher risk of developing the disorder themselves. While having a family member with schizophrenia does not guarantee that an individual will also develop the condition, genetics can certainly play a significant role in predisposing someone to schizophrenia.

In addition to genetic factors, environmental influences can also contribute to the development of schizophrenia. Traumatic life events, such as childhood abuse, neglect, or exposure to violence, can increase the risk of developing schizophrenia. Substance abuse, particularly during adolescence when the brain is still developing, has also been linked to an increased risk of developing the disorder.

Neurochemical imbalances in the brain are another potential cause of schizophrenia. Research has shown that individuals with schizophrenia may have abnormalities in the levels of certain neurotransmitters, such as dopamine and glutamate, which play a key role in regulating mood, cognition, and behavior.

These imbalances can disrupt the brain's ability to process information and may contribute to the development of schizophrenia.

While the exact causes of schizophrenia remain unknown, it is clear that a combination of genetic, environmental, and neurochemical factors all play a role in the development of the disorder. By understanding these potential causes, individuals and their families can work with healthcare professionals to develop effective treatment plans and strategies for managing the challenges associated with schizophrenia. It is important to remember that schizophrenia is a treatable condition, and with the right support and resources, individuals with schizophrenia can lead fulfilling and productive lives.

Diagnosis and Treatment Options

Diagnosing schizophrenia can be a complex and challenging process. It is essential for individuals and their families to be aware of the common symptoms of the disorder, which may include hallucinations, delusions, disorganized thinking, and social withdrawal.

If you or a loved one is experiencing these symptoms, it is crucial to seek help from a qualified mental health professional for a proper diagnosis.

Once a diagnosis of schizophrenia has been made, it is important to explore the various treatment options available. Medications, such as antipsychotic drugs, are often prescribed to help manage symptoms and improve overall functioning. It is essential for individuals and their families to work closely with a healthcare provider to find the right medication and dosage that works best for them.

In addition to medication, therapy can also be a valuable treatment option for individuals with schizophrenia. Cognitive-behavioral therapy (CBT) and family therapy are commonly used to help individuals better understand their condition and develop coping strategies. Therapy can also help families better understand and support their loved one with schizophrenia.

How To Manage Schizophrenia

It is crucial for individuals with schizophrenia and their families to work together to create a comprehensive treatment plan that addresses both the physical and emotional aspects of the disorder. Regular check-ins with healthcare providers, open communication, and a willingness to make adjustments to the treatment plan as needed are all important components of managing schizophrenia effectively.

While managing schizophrenia can be challenging, it is essential for individuals and their families to remain hopeful and dedicated to finding the right combination of treatments that work best for them. With the right support and resources, individuals with schizophrenia can lead fulfilling and productive lives. Remember, you are not alone in this journey, and there is help available to guide you through the challenges of living with schizophrenia.

How To Manage Schizophrenia

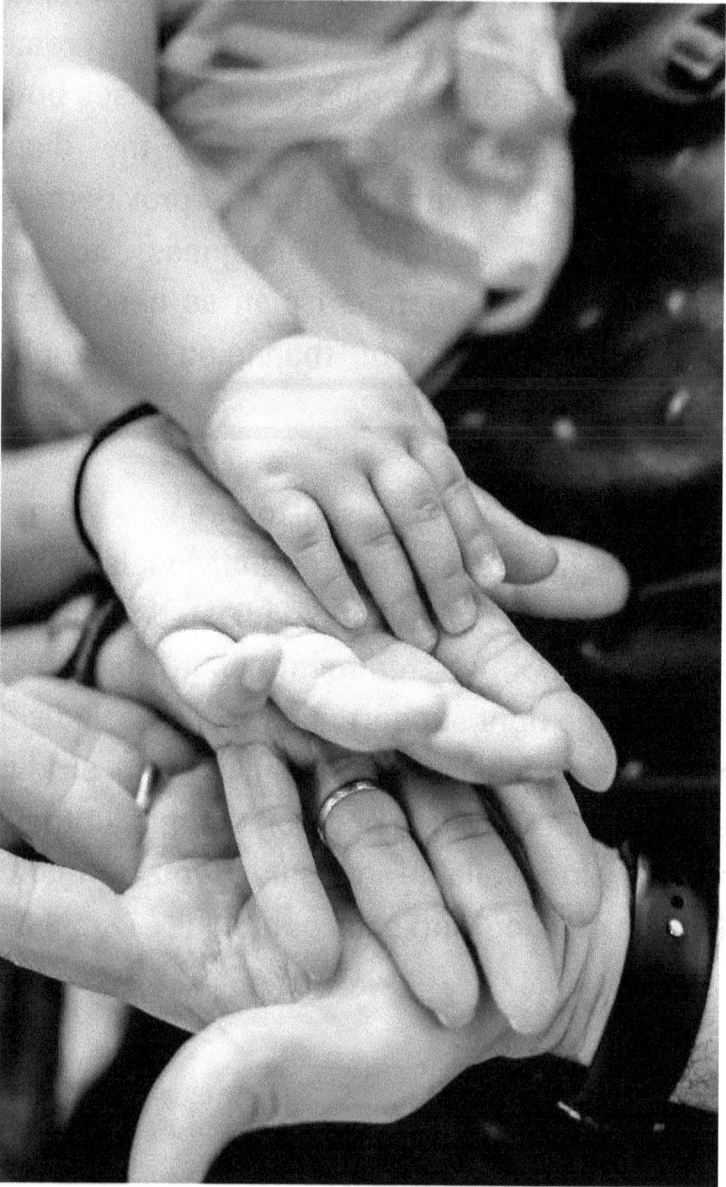

A Family's Guide to Navigating the Challenges

Chapter 2

Supporting a Loved One with Schizophrenia

Communicating Effectively

Communicating effectively is a crucial component in managing schizophrenia. People who have schizophrenia and their family members must understand the importance of clear and open communication to navigate the challenges that come with this mental illness. By learning effective communication strategies, both parties can ensure that their needs are met and that they are able to support each other in the best way possible.

One key aspect of communicating effectively is active listening. People who have schizophrenia may struggle to express themselves clearly due to their symptoms, so it is important for family members to listen attentively and show empathy. By giving their full attention and validating the person's feelings, family members can create a safe and supportive environment for meaningful conversations.

In addition to active listening, it is essential for both parties to be honest and open in their communication. People who have schizophrenia may have difficulty trusting others, so it is important for family members to be transparent and reliable in their interactions.

By being honest about their own feelings and concerns, family members can build trust and strengthen their relationship with their loved one who has schizophrenia.

Another important aspect of effective communication is using clear and simple language. People who have schizophrenia may have difficulty processing complex information, so it is important for family members to communicate in a way that is easy to understand. By using simple language and avoiding jargon, family members can ensure that their messages are received and understood accurately.

Overall, effective communication is key to managing schizophrenia and supporting both the person who has the illness and their family members.

By practicing active listening, honesty, and clarity in their interactions, people who have schizophrenia and their family members can strengthen their relationship and work together to navigate the challenges of living with this mental illness.

Providing Emotional Support

Providing emotional support to a loved one with schizophrenia is crucial in helping them navigate the challenges of the condition. It is important for family members to understand the emotional toll that schizophrenia can take on their loved one, and to offer them the support and understanding they need. Here are some tips and strategies for providing emotional support to someone with schizophrenia.

One important aspect of providing emotional support is to listen to your loved one without judgment. People with schizophrenia may experience hallucinations or delusions that can be frightening or confusing, and it is important to provide a safe space for them to talk about their experiences. By listening attentively and without judgment, you can help your loved one feel validated and understood.

Another way to provide emotional support is to help your loved one manage their stress and anxiety. Schizophrenia can be a highly stressful condition, and it is important to help your loved one find healthy coping mechanisms to deal with their emotions.

Encouraging them to engage in activities that they enjoy, such as exercise or creative hobbies, can help them to relax and de-stress.

It is also important to be patient and understanding with your loved one. Schizophrenia can be a complex and challenging condition, and it may take time for your loved one to come to terms with their diagnosis and learn to manage their symptoms. By being patient and supportive, you can help them to feel more confident in their ability to cope with the challenges of schizophrenia.

Finally, it is important to take care of yourself as well. Supporting a loved one with schizophrenia can be emotionally draining, and it is important to prioritize your own mental health and well-being.

Seeking support from other family members, friends, or a therapist can help you to cope with the challenges of supporting someone with schizophrenia, and ensure that you are able to provide the best possible support to your loved one.

Encouraging Treatment Adherence

Encouraging treatment adherence is crucial in managing schizophrenia effectively. People with schizophrenia may struggle with adhering to their treatment plan due to various reasons such as medication side effects, stigma surrounding mental health, and lack of insight into their condition. However, it is important for both the individual with schizophrenia and their family members to work together to prioritize treatment adherence for better long-term outcomes.

One way to encourage treatment adherence is by creating a supportive and understanding environment. Family members can play a significant role in helping their loved one with schizophrenia stay on track with their treatment plan.

By providing encouragement, understanding, and practical support, family members can help reduce the barriers to adherence that their loved one may face.

Education is another key component in encouraging treatment adherence. It is important for both the person with schizophrenia and their family members to have a good understanding of the benefits of treatment and the consequences of non-adherence. By educating themselves about the condition and treatment options, they can make more informed decisions and work together to develop a plan that is manageable and effective.

Regular communication between the person with schizophrenia, their family members, and healthcare providers is essential for successful treatment adherence. By keeping open lines of communication, all parties can stay informed about the progress of treatment, address any concerns or challenges that may arise, and make adjustments to the treatment plan as needed. This collaborative approach can help ensure that the individual with schizophrenia receives the support they need to adhere to their treatment plan.

Lastly, setting realistic goals and celebrating small victories can help motivate the person with schizophrenia to stay committed to their treatment plan. By acknowledging the efforts made and progress achieved, both the individual with schizophrenia and their family members can feel encouraged and motivated to continue working towards better management of the condition. Encouraging treatment adherence is a team effort that requires patience, understanding, and support from all parties involved.

Setting Boundaries

Setting boundaries is crucial when it comes to managing schizophrenia within a family dynamic. People who have schizophrenia and their families often struggle with establishing healthy boundaries that promote well-being and reduce stress.

By clearly defining limits and expectations, both parties can better navigate the challenges that come with the illness.

One way to set boundaries is to communicate openly and honestly about individual needs and limitations. People with schizophrenia may require more support and understanding from their families, while family members may need to establish boundaries to protect their own well-being. It is important to have ongoing conversations about what is and isn't acceptable behavior and to respect each other's boundaries.

Another important aspect of setting boundaries is to establish a routine that works for everyone involved. This can help reduce stress and uncertainty, which are common triggers for schizophrenia symptoms. By creating a structured environment with clear expectations, families can better support their loved ones with schizophrenia and maintain their own mental health.

It is also essential to recognize when boundaries are being crossed and to address the issue promptly and assertively. People with schizophrenia may struggle to understand social cues and boundaries, so it is important for family members to communicate clearly and consistently.

By setting firm boundaries and enforcing them consistently, families can help their loved ones with schizophrenia understand what is and isn't acceptable behavior.

Overall, setting boundaries is a key component of managing schizophrenia within a family. By communicating openly, establishing routines, and addressing boundary violations promptly, people with schizophrenia and their families can create a supportive and healthy environment that promotes well-being for everyone involved.

It may take time and effort to find the right balance, but by working together and respecting each other's needs, families can navigate the challenges of schizophrenia with greater ease.

How To Manage Schizophrenia

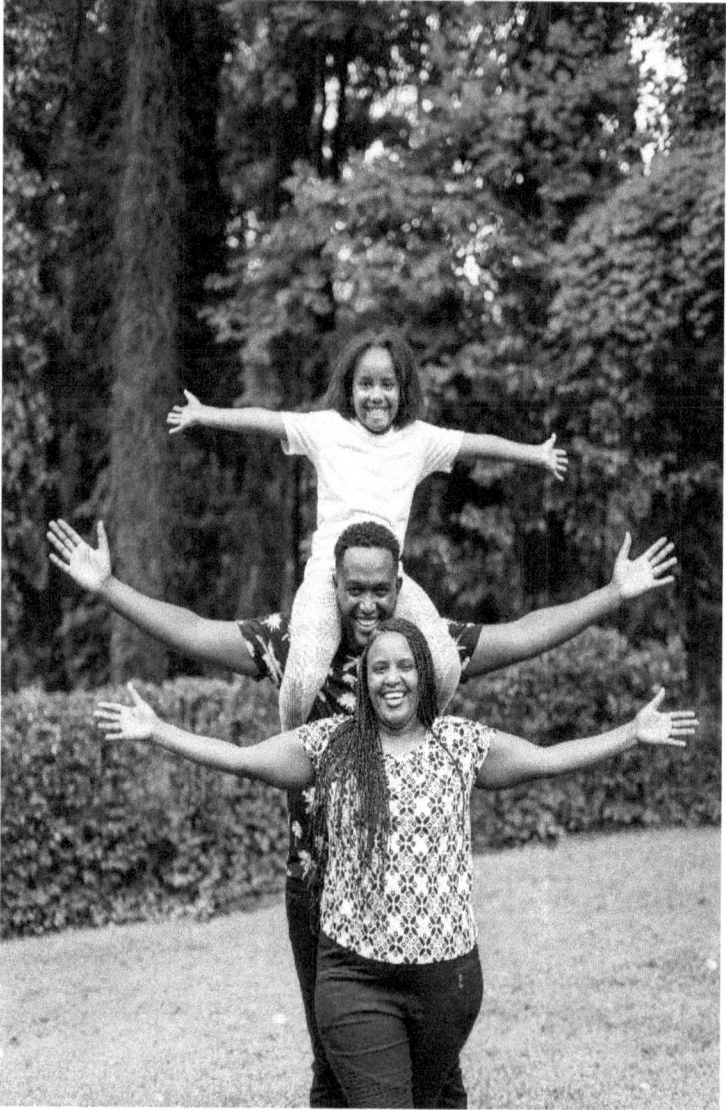

A Family's Guide to Navigating the Challenges

Chapter 3

Navigating Challenges as a Family

Dealing with Stigma

Dealing with the stigma surrounding schizophrenia can be one of the most challenging aspects of managing the condition. Many people hold misconceptions and stereotypes about schizophrenia, which can lead to discrimination and prejudice against individuals who have been diagnosed with the disorder. It is important for both people who have schizophrenia and their families to learn how to navigate and cope with this stigma in order to live fulfilling and empowered lives.

One of the first steps in dealing with stigma is education. It is crucial for individuals and their families to educate themselves about schizophrenia and the realities of living with the condition.

By understanding the symptoms, causes, and treatment options for schizophrenia, individuals can better advocate for themselves and challenge misconceptions when they arise.

Education can also help individuals build a strong support system of friends, family, and healthcare professionals who understand and respect their experiences.

Another important aspect of dealing with stigma is self-empowerment. People who have schizophrenia and their families should work to build self-confidence and resilience in the face of discrimination. This can involve setting boundaries with others, practicing self-care, and seeking out positive and supportive relationships.

By taking control of their own narratives and advocating for their needs, individuals can begin to break down the barriers of stigma and discrimination.

In addition to education and self-empowerment, individuals and their families can also work to challenge stigma on a broader societal level. This can involve participating in advocacy efforts, sharing personal stories, and promoting awareness and understanding of schizophrenia in their communities. By speaking out against stigma and discrimination, individuals can help to create a more accepting and inclusive society for all those affected by schizophrenia.

Overall, dealing with stigma is a complex and ongoing process for individuals and their families. By prioritizing education, self-empowerment, and advocacy, individuals can begin to challenge misconceptions and build a more supportive environment for themselves and others living with schizophrenia. It is important for individuals to remember that they are not defined by their diagnosis and that they deserve to be treated with dignity and respect. By working together to address stigma, individuals and their families can create a more compassionate and understanding world for all those affected by schizophrenia.

Managing Financial Strain

Managing financial strain can be a significant challenge for individuals and families affected by schizophrenia. The costs associated with treatment, medications, therapy, and other necessary support services can quickly add up, putting a strain on financial resources. It is important for individuals and families to create a financial plan to help manage these costs and alleviate some of the stress that comes with them.

One way to manage financial strain is to explore available resources and support services that can help offset some of the costs associated with schizophrenia treatment. Many communities offer financial assistance programs, support groups, and other resources that can help individuals and families manage the financial burden of schizophrenia. It is important to reach out to local organizations and healthcare providers to learn more about these resources and how to access them.

Another important aspect of managing financial strain is to create a budget and stick to it. By carefully tracking expenses and income, individuals and families can identify areas where costs can be reduced or eliminated.

This may involve cutting back on non-essential expenses, finding ways to save money on medications or treatment, or exploring alternative sources of income.

It is also important to communicate openly and honestly with healthcare providers about financial concerns. They may be able to provide guidance on ways to reduce costs, access financial assistance programs, or find alternative treatment options that are more affordable.

By working together with healthcare providers, individuals and families can develop a plan that addresses both the medical and financial aspects of managing schizophrenia.

Finally, it is important for individuals and families to prioritize self-care and mental health during times of financial strain. Stress and anxiety about money can exacerbate symptoms of schizophrenia, making it even more important to practice self-care techniques such as mindfulness, exercise, and relaxation exercises. By taking care of both their financial and mental health, individuals and families can better navigate the challenges of managing schizophrenia.

Balancing Caregiving Responsibilities

Balancing caregiving responsibilities when a loved one has schizophrenia can be a challenging and overwhelming task. It is important for both the individual with schizophrenia and their family members to work together to find a balance that works for everyone involved.

This subchapter will provide tips and strategies for managing caregiving responsibilities while also taking care of oneself.

One important aspect of balancing caregiving responsibilities is communication. It is crucial for family members to openly communicate with one another and with the individual with schizophrenia about their needs and concerns. Setting boundaries and expectations can help prevent burnout and resentment. It is also important to listen actively and empathetically to the needs of the individual with schizophrenia, as their perspective is crucial in finding a balance that works for everyone.

Another key aspect of balancing caregiving responsibilities is self-care. It is essential for family members to take care of themselves both physically and emotionally in order to effectively care for their loved one with schizophrenia.

This may involve setting aside time for relaxation and hobbies, seeking support from friends and other family members, and attending therapy or support groups. Taking breaks and prioritizing self-care is not selfish, but rather necessary for maintaining a healthy caregiving relationship.

In addition to communication and self-care, it is important for family members to educate themselves about schizophrenia and its management. Understanding the symptoms, treatment options, and potential challenges associated with schizophrenia can help family members better support their loved one and navigate the caregiving responsibilities. Seeking information from mental health professionals, support groups, and reputable resources can help family members feel more confident in their caregiving role.

Lastly, seeking professional help and support is crucial in balancing caregiving responsibilities. Family members should not hesitate to reach out to mental health professionals, such as therapists, psychiatrists, and social workers, for guidance and support. Additionally, joining support groups for caregivers of individuals with schizophrenia can provide a sense of community and understanding. By working together and seeking help when needed, family members can effectively balance their caregiving responsibilities and provide the best possible support for their loved one with schizophrenia.

Seeking Support for Yourself

Seeking support for yourself is crucial when you or a loved one is living with schizophrenia. It is important to recognize that managing schizophrenia can be overwhelming at times, and seeking support from others can make a significant difference in your overall well-being.

Whether you are someone living with schizophrenia or a family member supporting a loved one, reaching out for help is a sign of strength, not weakness.

One of the first steps in seeking support for yourself is to educate yourself about schizophrenia and its symptoms. Understanding the nature of the illness can help you better navigate the challenges that come with managing schizophrenia. There are many resources available, such as books, websites, and support groups, that can provide valuable information and guidance on how to cope with the symptoms of schizophrenia.

In addition to educating yourself about schizophrenia, it is also important to find a support system that you can turn to for help. This may include family members, friends, healthcare professionals, or support groups specifically for individuals and families affected by schizophrenia.

Having a strong support system can provide you with emotional support, practical assistance, and a sense of community that can help you feel less isolated in your journey.

It is also important to prioritize self-care when seeking support for yourself. Managing schizophrenia can be draining both emotionally and physically, so it is essential to take care of yourself by eating well, getting enough sleep, exercising regularly, and engaging in activities that bring you joy and relaxation. Practicing self-care can help you maintain your overall well-being and resilience in the face of the challenges that come with managing schizophrenia.

Finally, remember that seeking support for yourself is not a sign of weakness, but rather a necessary step in managing schizophrenia effectively. By reaching out for help, you are taking an active role in your own well-being and showing that you are committed to your own recovery. Remember that you are not alone in this journey, and there are many resources and people available to support you every step of the way.

How To Manage Schizophrenia

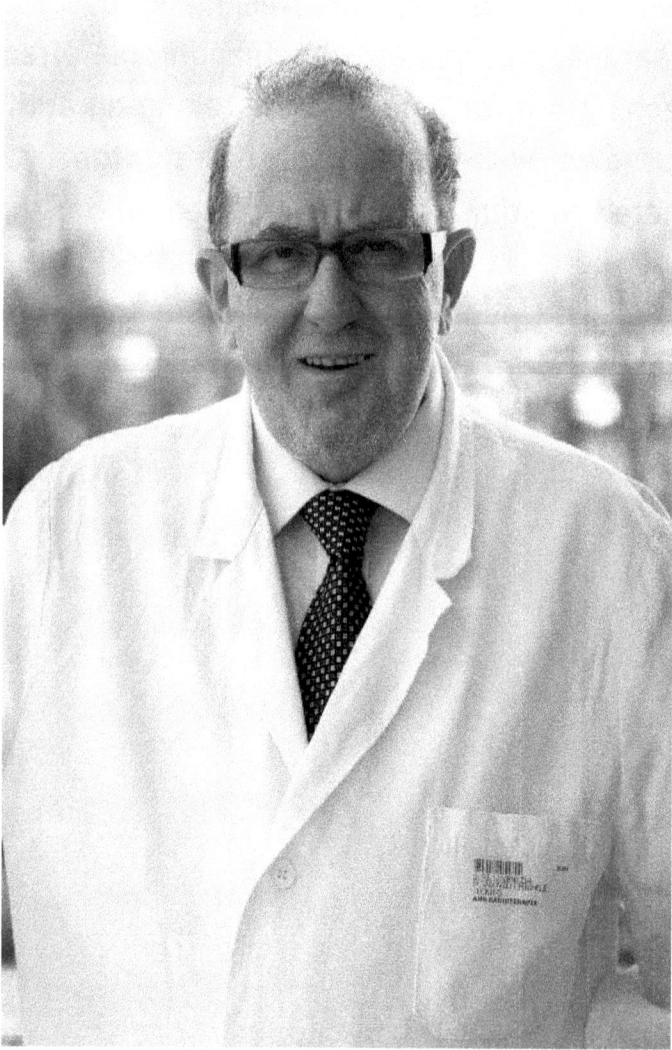

Chapter 4

Building a Strong Support System

Connecting with Mental Health Professionals

Connecting with mental health professionals is crucial for individuals living with schizophrenia and their families. These professionals have the expertise and experience to provide the necessary support and guidance to navigate the challenges that come with managing this complex mental illness.

By establishing a strong relationship with mental health professionals, individuals and their families can work together to develop a comprehensive treatment plan that addresses both the physical and emotional aspects of schizophrenia.

When seeking out mental health professionals, it is important to find a team that is knowledgeable about schizophrenia and has experience working with individuals who have this condition. This may include psychiatrists, psychologists, social workers, and other professionals who specialize in mental health care.

It is also important to find professionals who are compassionate, patient, and willing to work collaboratively with individuals and their families to develop a personalized treatment plan.

In addition to finding the right professionals, it is important to establish open and honest communication with them. This includes being transparent about symptoms, concerns, and treatment preferences.

By being proactive in communicating with mental health professionals, individuals and their families can ensure that they are receiving the best possible care and support.

Mental health professionals can also provide valuable resources and information to help individuals and their families better understand schizophrenia and how to effectively manage symptoms. This may include educational materials, support groups, and referrals to other healthcare providers.

By taking advantage of these resources, individuals and their families can gain a deeper understanding of schizophrenia and learn strategies for coping with the challenges it presents.

Overall, connecting with mental health professionals is an essential part of managing schizophrenia. By working together with a team of knowledgeable and compassionate professionals, individuals and their families can develop a comprehensive treatment plan that addresses their unique needs and challenges. Through open communication, collaboration, and access to valuable resources, individuals living with schizophrenia can improve their quality of life and achieve better mental health outcomes.

Joining Support Groups

Joining support groups can be an invaluable resource for individuals living with schizophrenia and their families. These groups provide a safe space for sharing experiences, coping strategies, and emotional support with others who understand the challenges of living with this condition. By connecting with others who are going through similar struggles, individuals can feel less isolated and more understood, which can help to alleviate feelings of loneliness and stigma.

Support groups also offer practical advice and information on managing schizophrenia symptoms, navigating the healthcare system, and accessing resources and services in the community. Members can learn from each other's experiences and gain insights into different treatment options, therapy techniques, and self-care practices that may be helpful in managing the condition.

By participating in these groups, individuals can build a network of support that can help them feel more empowered and capable of coping with the challenges of living with schizophrenia.

In addition to the emotional and practical support that support groups provide, they can also be a source of hope and inspiration for individuals and their families. Hearing success stories from others who have learned to manage their symptoms, build fulfilling lives, and overcome obstacles can instill a sense of optimism and motivation in those who may be struggling.

By seeing that recovery is possible and that there is a community of people who understand and care, individuals can feel more hopeful about their own journey towards wellness.

Support groups can also help individuals and their families develop coping skills, communication strategies, and problem-solving techniques that can improve their relationships and enhance their quality of life. By learning how to communicate effectively, set boundaries, and practice empathy and understanding, family members can create a more supportive and harmonious environment for their loved one with schizophrenia.

Additionally, individuals can gain tools for managing stress, anxiety, and other emotions that may arise in their daily lives, which can help to reduce the impact of symptoms and improve overall well-being.

Overall, joining a support group can be a transformative experience for individuals living with schizophrenia and their families. By connecting with others who understand their struggles, sharing experiences and resources, and learning coping strategies and skills, individuals can feel more empowered, supported, and hopeful on their journey towards recovery and wellness.

Support groups can provide a sense of belonging, understanding, and community that can make a significant difference in the lives of those affected by schizophrenia.

Educating Yourself about Schizophrenia

One of the most important steps in managing schizophrenia is to educate yourself about the condition. Understanding the symptoms, causes, and treatment options can help both individuals with schizophrenia and their families navigate the challenges that come with the disorder.

By learning more about schizophrenia, you can better advocate for yourself or your loved one and make informed decisions about treatment and support.

Schizophrenia is a complex and often misunderstood mental health condition that affects how a person thinks, feels, and behaves. Common symptoms include delusions, hallucinations, disorganized thinking, and difficulty focusing or paying attention.

It is important to recognize that schizophrenia is a brain disorder and not a character flaw or personal weakness. By educating yourself about the biological basis of schizophrenia, you can reduce stigma and better support yourself or your loved one.

There are many resources available to help you learn more about schizophrenia. Books, websites, support groups, and mental health professionals can provide valuable information and guidance. It is important to seek out reliable sources of information and avoid misinformation or stereotypes about schizophrenia. By educating yourself from reputable sources, you can gain a deeper understanding of the condition and how to effectively manage it.

In addition to learning about schizophrenia, it is important to stay informed about treatment options and support services. Medication, therapy, and lifestyle changes can all play a role in managing the symptoms of schizophrenia and improving quality of life. By working closely with mental health professionals, individuals with schizophrenia and their families can develop a comprehensive treatment plan that addresses their unique needs and goals.

Overall, educating yourself about schizophrenia is a crucial step in managing the condition and promoting recovery. By gaining knowledge and understanding about the disorder, individuals with schizophrenia and their families can advocate for themselves, access appropriate treatment, and build a strong support network.

By taking an active role in learning about schizophrenia, you can empower yourself to navigate the challenges of the condition and live a fulfilling life.

Fostering Resilience in Your Family

In the journey of managing schizophrenia, fostering resilience in your family is crucial to navigating the challenges that come with the condition. Building resilience within your family unit can help you all better cope with the ups and downs that may arise, and ultimately strengthen your bond as a support system for each other.

One way to foster resilience in your family is by promoting open and honest communication. Encouraging dialogue about thoughts, feelings, and experiences related to schizophrenia can help create a safe space for everyone to share their concerns and seek support. By openly discussing the challenges and victories that come with managing schizophrenia, you can build a sense of solidarity and understanding within your family.

Another important aspect of fostering resilience in your family is creating a support network. This can include reaching out to mental health professionals, support groups, and other resources that can provide guidance and assistance. By connecting with others who have experience in managing schizophrenia, you can gain valuable insights and advice that can help strengthen your family's resilience.

It is also important to practice self-care within your family unit. Managing schizophrenia can be emotionally and physically draining, so taking time to prioritize your own well-being is essential. Encouraging each family member to engage in activities that bring them joy and relaxation can help build resilience and prevent burnout.

Lastly, fostering resilience in your family involves cultivating a sense of hope and optimism for the future. By setting realistic goals and celebrating small victories along the way, you can build a sense of positive momentum that can help you all navigate the challenges of managing schizophrenia together.

Remember, you are not alone in this journey, and by fostering resilience within your family, you can support each other through the highs and lows that come with living with schizophrenia.

How To Manage Schizophrenia

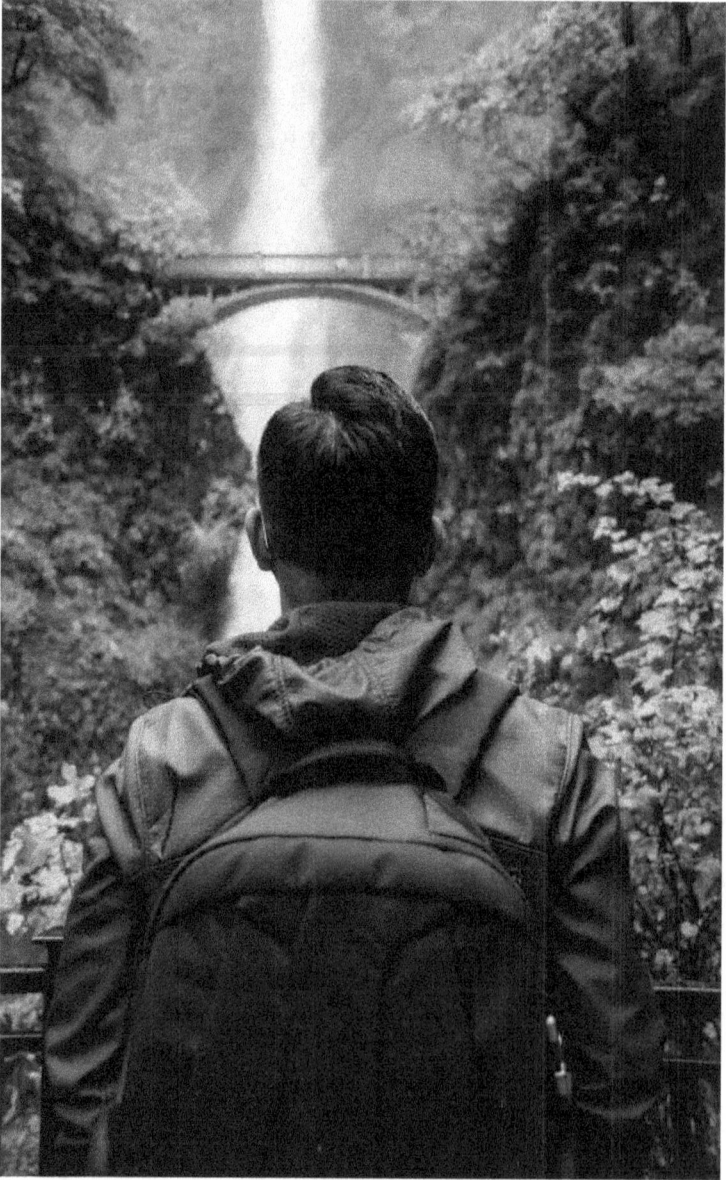

A Family's Guide to Navigating the Challenges

Chapter 5

Self-Care for Family Members

Managing Stress and Burnout

Managing stress and burnout is crucial for individuals living with schizophrenia and their families. The daily challenges and uncertainties can take a toll on mental and emotional well-being, making it essential to have effective strategies in place to cope with stress and prevent burnout. In this subchapter, we will explore practical tips and techniques to help you navigate the ups and downs of managing schizophrenia.

One of the first steps in managing stress and burnout is to prioritize self-care. It's important for individuals with schizophrenia and their families to take time for themselves and engage in activities that promote relaxation and rejuvenation.

This could include practicing mindfulness, exercise, hobbies, or spending time with loved ones. By taking care of yourself, you'll be better equipped to handle the challenges that come with managing schizophrenia.

Another helpful strategy for managing stress is to establish a support system. Surrounding yourself with friends, family, or support groups can provide a sense of community and understanding during difficult times. It's important to have a network of people who can offer guidance, encouragement, and a listening ear when needed. By building a support system, you can reduce feelings of isolation and find comfort in knowing that you're not alone in your journey.

Setting boundaries is another important aspect of managing stress and preventing burnout. It's essential to recognize your limits and communicate them to others. This could include setting boundaries around work, relationships, or responsibilities to avoid becoming overwhelmed. By establishing healthy boundaries, you can create a sense of balance and control in your life, reducing the risk of burnout.

Lastly, seeking professional help is a vital step in managing stress and burnout. Whether it's therapy, counseling, or medication management, it's important to prioritize your mental health and well-being. A mental health professional can provide you with the necessary tools and resources to cope with stress, manage symptoms, and prevent burnout. Remember, it's okay to ask for help and seek support when needed. By taking proactive steps to manage stress and burnout, you can navigate the challenges of schizophrenia with resilience and strength.

Prioritizing Your Own Mental Health

When you or a loved one is living with schizophrenia, it's easy to get caught up in the day-to-day challenges of managing symptoms and navigating the healthcare system. However, it's essential to remember that taking care of your own mental health is just as important as managing the symptoms of the illness. Prioritizing your mental health can help you and your loved one cope better with the challenges of living with schizophrenia.

One way to prioritize your mental health is to make time for self-care activities that help you relax and unwind. Whether it's taking a walk in nature, practicing meditation, or engaging in a hobby you enjoy, finding ways to de-stress and recharge can have a positive impact on your mental well-being. Remember, it's okay to take a break from caregiving responsibilities to focus on yourself.

Another important aspect of prioritizing your mental health is seeking support from others who understand what you're going through. Connecting with support groups for people living with schizophrenia or their families can provide a sense of community and understanding that can be invaluable in times of need. Talking to others who are going through similar experiences can help you feel less alone and more supported.

It's also crucial to practice good self-care habits, such as getting enough sleep, eating a healthy diet, and exercising regularly. These simple habits can have a significant impact on your mental health and overall well-being.

Remember, taking care of yourself is not selfish – it's necessary for you to be able to continue supporting your loved one with schizophrenia.

In conclusion, prioritizing your own mental health is essential when you or a loved one is living with schizophrenia. By taking time for self-care activities, seeking support from others, and practicing good self-care habits, you can better cope with the challenges of managing the illness. Remember, you are not alone – there are resources and communities available to help you through this journey. Take care of yourself, so you can continue to support your loved one with schizophrenia.

Finding Time for Relaxation and Hobbies

Finding time for relaxation and hobbies can be a crucial aspect of managing schizophrenia. It is important for individuals with schizophrenia and their families to prioritize self-care and stress management in order to maintain overall well-being.

How To Manage Schizophrenia

Engaging in activities that bring joy and relaxation can help reduce symptoms and improve quality of life for those living with schizophrenia.

One way to make time for relaxation and hobbies is to create a schedule that includes designated time for self-care activities. This could include setting aside time each day for activities such as reading, painting, or taking a walk in nature.

By intentionally scheduling time for relaxation, individuals with schizophrenia can prioritize their mental health and reduce feelings of stress and anxiety.

It is also important for individuals with schizophrenia and their families to identify hobbies and activities that bring joy and fulfillment. Engaging in activities that provide a sense of accomplishment and satisfaction can help boost self-esteem and improve overall mental well-being. Whether it's gardening, cooking, or playing a musical instrument, finding a hobby that brings joy can be a powerful tool in managing schizophrenia.

In addition to finding time for relaxation and hobbies, it is important for individuals with schizophrenia to prioritize physical health as well. Regular exercise, healthy eating, and getting enough sleep can all play a role in managing symptoms of schizophrenia and improving overall well-being. By taking care of their physical health, individuals with schizophrenia can better manage stress and reduce symptoms.

Overall, finding time for relaxation and hobbies is an essential part of managing schizophrenia. By prioritizing self-care, engaging in fulfilling activities, and taking care of physical health, individuals with schizophrenia can improve their overall well-being and quality of life. It is important for individuals with schizophrenia and their families to work together to prioritize self-care and stress management in order to navigate the challenges of living with schizophrenia.

Seeking Help When Needed

Seeking help when needed is crucial for individuals with schizophrenia and their families. It is important to remember that schizophrenia is a serious mental health condition that requires professional support and guidance.

If you or a loved one is experiencing symptoms of schizophrenia, it is essential to seek help from a qualified mental health professional as soon as possible.

When seeking help for schizophrenia, it is important to find a healthcare provider who specializes in treating this condition. A psychiatrist or psychologist with experience in schizophrenia can provide the best care and support for individuals and families dealing with this challenging illness.

It is also important to communicate openly and honestly with your healthcare provider about your symptoms, concerns, and treatment preferences.

In addition to professional help, it is also important to seek support from family and friends. Having a strong support system can make a significant difference in managing schizophrenia. Family members and friends can provide emotional support, help with daily tasks, and offer encouragement during difficult times.

It is important to communicate openly with your loved ones about your needs and how they can support you in your journey towards recovery.

In some cases, individuals with schizophrenia may need additional support from community resources, such as support groups or mental health organizations.

These resources can provide valuable information, education, and support for individuals and families dealing with schizophrenia. It is important to reach out to these resources for help and guidance, as they can offer valuable insight and assistance in managing the challenges of schizophrenia.

Overall, seeking help when needed is essential for individuals with schizophrenia and their families. By reaching out to qualified healthcare professionals, building a strong support system, and utilizing community resources, individuals with schizophrenia can effectively manage their symptoms and work towards recovery. Remember, you are not alone in this journey, and there are resources available to help you navigate the challenges of schizophrenia.

How To Manage Schizophrenia

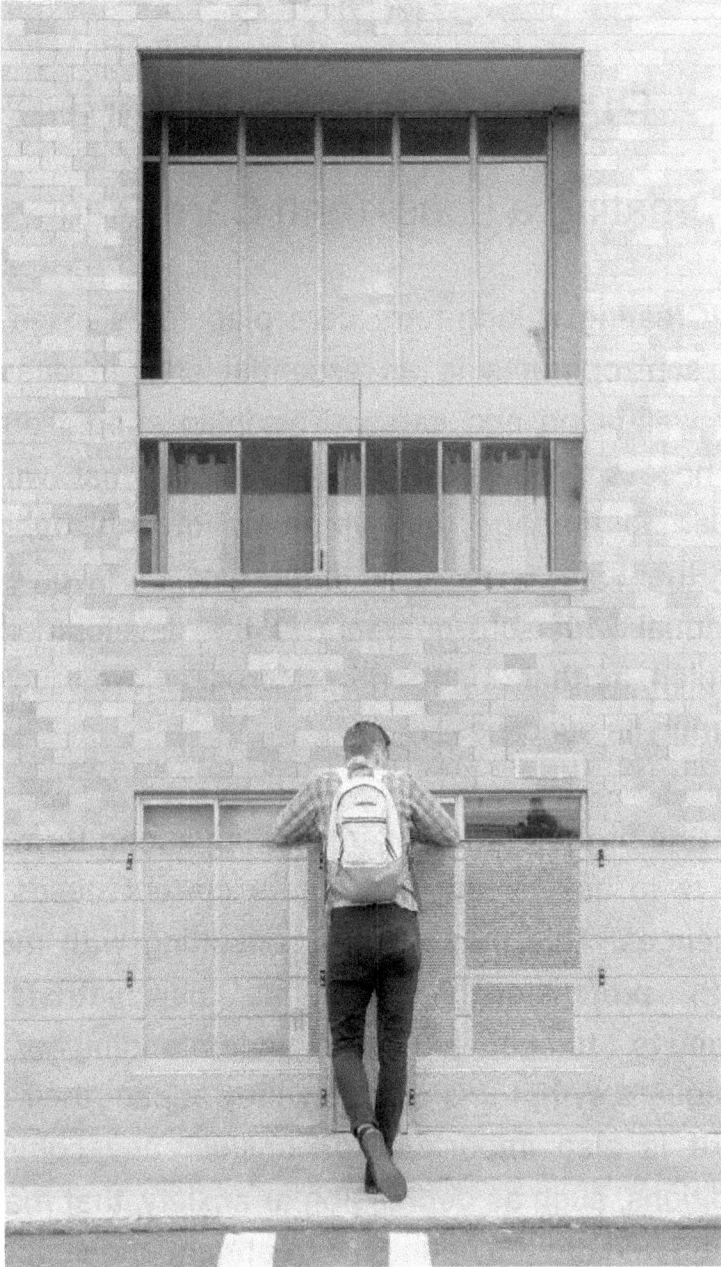

A Family's Guide to Navigating the Challenges

Chapter 6

Planning for the Future

Creating a Long-Term Care Plan

Creating a long-term care plan for a loved one with schizophrenia is an essential step in ensuring their well-being and safety. This plan should outline the necessary support and resources that will be needed to manage the symptoms of schizophrenia over the long term. It is important to involve the individual with schizophrenia in the development of this plan, as their input and preferences are crucial in ensuring its success.

One of the first steps in creating a long-term care plan is to assess the individual's current needs and challenges. This may involve consulting with mental health professionals, such as psychiatrists or therapists, to get a better understanding of the individual's symptoms and how they impact their daily life. It is also important to consider any comorbid conditions, such as depression or anxiety, that may be present and require additional treatment and support.

Once the individual's needs have been assessed, the next step is to identify the support and resources that will be needed to address these needs. This may include medication management, therapy, case management services, and support groups.

It is important to research and connect with local mental health resources in the community to ensure that the individual has access to the appropriate care and services.

In addition to professional support, it is also important to include family members and loved ones in the long-term care plan. Family members can provide valuable emotional support and assistance in managing the individual's symptoms. It is important to establish clear communication channels and boundaries within the family to ensure that everyone is on the same page and working towards the same goals.

Finally, it is important to regularly review and update the long-term care plan as needed. As the individual's symptoms and needs may change over time, it is important to be flexible and adaptable in adjusting the care plan to meet these changing needs. By creating a comprehensive long-term care plan, individuals with schizophrenia and their families can feel more confident and prepared in managing the challenges of this complex mental health condition.

Exploring Housing Options

When it comes to managing schizophrenia, one of the key factors to consider is finding suitable housing options that provide a safe and supportive environment for individuals with the condition. There are a variety of housing options available, ranging from independent living arrangements to more structured group homes or residential treatment facilities.

It's important for individuals and their families to carefully consider their needs and preferences when exploring housing options, as finding the right fit can greatly impact the individual's overall well-being and stability.

Independent living arrangements are a popular choice for individuals with schizophrenia who are able to live on their own with minimal support. These options can include renting an apartment or house, living with roommates, or even owning a home. While independent living can provide individuals with a sense of autonomy and freedom, it's important to ensure that the individual has access to necessary support services and resources to help them maintain their independence and manage their symptoms effectively.

For individuals who may require more support and structure in their living environment, group homes or residential treatment facilities can be a beneficial option. These types of housing options typically provide 24-hour staff support, medication management, therapy services, and socialization opportunities for residents.

While group homes and residential treatment facilities can be more restrictive in terms of rules and regulations, they can also offer a higher level of supervision and support for individuals who may struggle to live independently.

Another important consideration when exploring housing options for individuals with schizophrenia is the location of the housing facility. It's important to consider factors such as proximity to medical and mental health services, public transportation options, and community resources when selecting a housing option.

Being located near essential services and supports can make it easier for individuals with schizophrenia to access the care and resources they need to manage their symptoms and maintain their overall well-being.

Overall, exploring housing options for individuals with schizophrenia requires careful consideration of the individual's needs, preferences, and level of support required. By carefully evaluating the available options and selecting a housing arrangement that meets the individual's unique needs, individuals and their families can help to create a safe, stable, and supportive environment that promotes recovery and well-being.

Estate Planning and Legal Considerations

Estate planning is a crucial aspect to consider for individuals living with schizophrenia and their families. Planning for the future is essential to ensure that your loved one's assets and affairs are taken care of in the event of their incapacitation or passing. It is important to have a clear plan in place to protect their interests and provide for their financial and medical needs.

One of the key legal considerations in estate planning for individuals with schizophrenia is the establishment of a durable power of attorney. This legal document allows a trusted individual to make financial and medical decisions on behalf of the person living with schizophrenia in the event that they are unable to do so themselves.

It is important to choose someone who is knowledgeable about the individual's needs and wishes, and who can be trusted to act in their best interests.

Another important legal consideration in estate planning is the creation of a will. A will is a legal document that outlines how the individual's assets and possessions should be distributed after their passing. It is important to work with an experienced attorney to ensure that the will is legally valid and accurately reflects the individual's wishes. A will can help avoid disputes among family members and ensure that the individual's wishes are carried out as intended.

In addition to a power of attorney and a will, individuals with schizophrenia and their families may also want to consider setting up a trust. A trust is a legal arrangement that allows a designated trustee to hold and manage assets on behalf of the individual with schizophrenia. A trust can provide added protection for the individual's assets and ensure that they are used for their benefit.

Overall, estate planning and legal considerations are important aspects of managing schizophrenia and ensuring that the individual's needs are met both now and in the future.

By working with experienced legal professionals and carefully planning for the future, individuals with schizophrenia and their families can have peace of mind knowing that their affairs are in order and their interests are protected.

Advocating for Policy Changes in Mental Health Care

Advocating for Policy Changes in Mental Health Care is an important aspect of supporting loved ones with schizophrenia. As family members, it is crucial to understand the current state of mental health care policies and how they impact individuals with schizophrenia. By advocating for policy changes, we can ensure that our loved ones receive the best possible care and support in their journey towards recovery.

One way to advocate for policy changes is to stay informed about current mental health legislation and initiatives. By keeping up-to-date with local, state, and national policies, we can identify areas that need improvement and work towards creating positive change.

This may involve attending town hall meetings, contacting elected officials, and participating in advocacy groups that focus on mental health issues.

Another important aspect of advocating for policy changes is to share personal stories and experiences with schizophrenia. By raising awareness about the challenges faced by individuals with schizophrenia and their families, we can help policymakers understand the need for improved mental health care services. Personal stories have the power to humanize the issue and create empathy among decision-makers.

In addition to sharing personal stories, it is also important to collaborate with mental health professionals, advocacy organizations, and other stakeholders in the mental health care system. By working together, we can amplify our voices and create a unified front for policy change. Building strong partnerships with like-minded individuals and organizations can help us achieve our advocacy goals more effectively.

Overall, advocating for policy changes in mental health care is a crucial part of supporting loved ones with schizophrenia. By staying informed, sharing personal stories, and collaborating with others, we can make a positive impact on the mental health care system and ensure that individuals with schizophrenia receive the care and support they deserve. Together, we can work towards creating a more inclusive and supportive environment for those living with schizophrenia.

How To Manage Schizophrenia

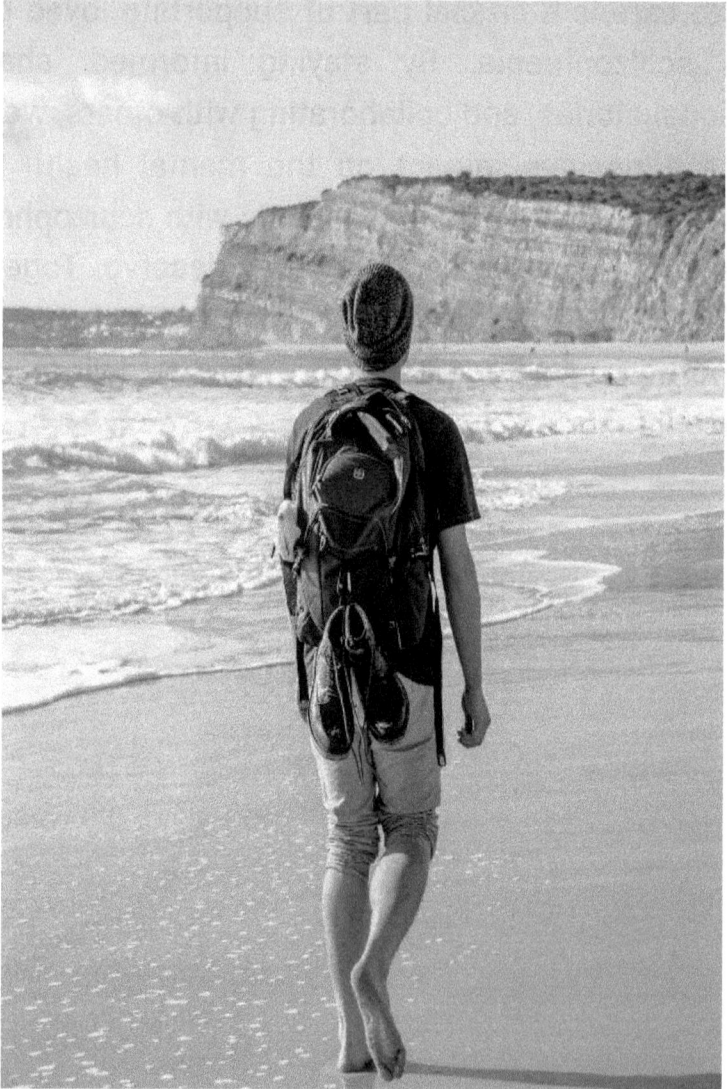

A Family's Guide to Navigating the Challenges

Chapter 7

Celebrating Victories and Milestones

Recognizing Progress and Achievements

When it comes to managing schizophrenia, it is important for both individuals with the disorder and their families to recognize and celebrate progress and achievements. Living with schizophrenia can be challenging, but it is essential to acknowledge the small victories along the way.

Whether it's successfully attending a therapy session, taking medication regularly, or even just getting out of bed in the morning, every accomplishment is a step in the right direction.

It can be easy to focus on the negative aspects of schizophrenia, such as symptoms and setbacks. However, by taking the time to acknowledge progress and achievements, individuals with schizophrenia and their families can build confidence and motivation to continue working towards recovery. Celebrating even the smallest victories can help to create a positive mindset and reinforce the idea that recovery is possible.

One way to recognize progress and achievements is to keep a journal or log of accomplishments. This can help individuals with schizophrenia and their families track their progress over time and reflect on how far they have come. Writing down achievements, no matter how small, can serve as a reminder of the hard work and dedication that has been put into managing the disorder.

Another way to recognize progress and achievements is to set goals and milestones. By breaking down larger tasks into smaller, more manageable steps, individuals with schizophrenia can track their progress and celebrate each milestone along the way.

Setting realistic goals can provide a sense of direction and purpose, and achieving these goals can boost self-esteem and confidence.

Overall, recognizing progress and achievements is an integral part of managing schizophrenia. By celebrating even the smallest victories, individuals with the disorder and their families can stay motivated and focused on their journey towards recovery. Remember, progress is not always linear, and setbacks may occur. However, by acknowledging achievements and staying positive, individuals with schizophrenia can continue to strive towards a fulfilling life.

Reflecting on Challenges Overcome

Living with schizophrenia can present many challenges for both the individual diagnosed with the disorder and their family members. However, it is important to take a moment to reflect on the challenges that have been overcome along the way. By acknowledging and celebrating these victories, it can help to build resilience and provide motivation for facing future obstacles.

How To Manage Schizophrenia

One of the most common challenges faced by individuals with schizophrenia is stigma and discrimination. Many people hold misconceptions about the disorder, leading to feelings of shame and isolation. However, by actively challenging these stereotypes and educating others about schizophrenia, individuals and their families can help to break down barriers and promote understanding and acceptance.

Another significant challenge that individuals with schizophrenia may face is managing symptoms such as hallucinations and delusions. This can be a daunting task, but with the support of mental health professionals and loved ones, it is possible to learn coping strategies and techniques to help manage these symptoms. By working together as a team, individuals can develop a personalized treatment plan that addresses their specific needs and goals.

In addition to symptom management, individuals with schizophrenia may also struggle with medication adherence. It can be difficult to stay on top of a medication regimen, especially when side effects are present.

However, by establishing a routine and utilizing tools such as pill organizers or reminder apps, individuals can increase their chances of successfully adhering to their treatment plan. Family members can also play a supportive role by offering reminders and encouragement.

Reflecting on the challenges that have been overcome can provide a sense of empowerment and hope for the future. By recognizing the progress that has been made, individuals and their families can build confidence in their ability to navigate the complexities of living with schizophrenia.

Through open communication, mutual support, and a willingness to seek help when needed, it is possible to overcome challenges and thrive despite the obstacles that may arise.

Finding Joy and Hope in the Journey of Supporting a Loved One with Schizophrenia

Supporting a loved one with schizophrenia can be a challenging journey, but it is important to remember that there is hope and joy to be found along the way. It is crucial to approach the situation with understanding and compassion, as schizophrenia is a complex and often misunderstood mental illness.

By educating yourself about the symptoms and treatment options, you can better support your loved one in their journey towards recovery.

Finding joy in the journey of supporting a loved one with schizophrenia can come from small moments of connection and progress. Celebrate the victories, no matter how small they may seem, and focus on the positive aspects of your loved one's journey. This can help both you and your loved one stay motivated and hopeful for the future. Remember that recovery is a process, and setbacks are a normal part of the journey.

It is also important to take care of yourself as a caregiver. Supporting a loved one with schizophrenia can be emotionally draining, so be sure to prioritize your own mental health and well-being. Seek out support from other caregivers or mental health professionals, and make time for self-care activities that bring you joy and relaxation. By taking care of yourself, you will be better equipped to support your loved one in their journey towards recovery.

Finding hope in the journey of supporting a loved one with schizophrenia can come from staying informed about the latest research and treatment options. While schizophrenia is a chronic condition, there are many effective treatments available that can help your loved one manage their symptoms and lead a fulfilling life.

By staying proactive and advocating for your loved one's needs, you can help them navigate the challenges of living with schizophrenia and find hope for the future.

In conclusion, supporting a loved one with schizophrenia can be a difficult and emotional journey, but it is also a journey filled with moments of joy and hope. By approaching the situation with understanding, compassion, and a focus on the positive aspects of your loved one's journey, you can help them navigate the challenges of living with schizophrenia and find hope for the future.

Remember to take care of yourself as a caregiver, stay informed about the latest research and treatment options, and celebrate the small victories along the way. With your love and support, your loved one can find hope and joy in their journey towards recovery.

Author Notes & Acknowledgments

First and foremost, I would like to express my deepest gratitude to the people who inspired and supported me throughout the journey of writing this book. This project would not have been possible without their unwavering belief in me and their invaluable contributions.

To my wife, thank you for your constant encouragement and understanding. Your love and support have been my anchor during the challenging times of researching and writing this book. Your belief in my ability to make a difference in people's lives has been my driving force.

I would also like to disclose that this book contains some renewed artificial intelligence-generated content. I really appreciate very recent technological innovation by outstanding scientists and of course our reader's understanding.

Lastly, I want to express my deepest gratitude to the readers of this book. I sincerely hope the strategies and methods outlined within these pages will provide you with the knowledge and tools needed to truly make your life much better. Your commitment to seeking any good solutions and willingness to explore multiple methods is commendable.

Author Bio

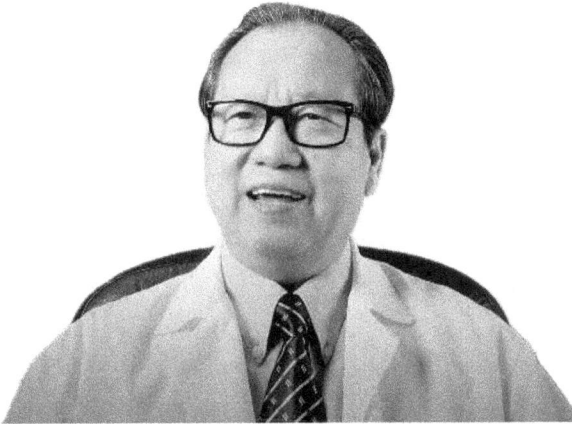

Johnson Wu earned his MD in 1982. With over 40 years of clinical experience, he has worked in hospitals in Zhejiang and Shanghai, China, as well as the Royal Marsden Hospital (part of Imperial College) in London, UK. Upon the recommendation of Sir Aaron Klug, the president of The Royal Society and a Nobel Prize winner in Chemistry, Dr. Wu was honorably awarded a British Royal Society Fellowship. He has published over 100 medical books in many countries and currently practices medicine in Canada.

www.ingramcontent.com/pod-product-compliance
Lightning Source LLC
Chambersburg PA
CBHW070028030426
42335CB00017B/2339